BDSM: Dirty Talk 101

A Beginners Guide To Sexy, Naughty & Hot Dirty Talking To Help Spice Up Your Love Life

Maxwell Diamond

Copyright © 2018 Maxwell Diamond

All rights reserved.

Although the author and publisher have made every effort to ensure that the information presented in this book was correct at the present time, the author and publisher do not assume and hereby disclaim any liability to any party for any loss, damage, or disruption caused by errors or omissions, whether such errors or omissions result from negligence, accident, or any other cause.

ISBN: 9781790250424

BDSM: Dirty Talk 101

CONTENTS

Introduction 8

   So what is BDSM? 9

   What is the difference between a Kink and a Fetish? 10

   Paraphilias 10

   Consent, Safety and Safe Words 11

   A list of Safe Words 12

   Non Verbal Safe Words 13

   Traffic Light System 13

   Pain vs. Pleasure 14

   Common misconceptions about BDSM 15

Types of Dirty Talk 17

   Playful 17

   Complementary 17

   Degrading 18

   Personal 18

In Relation To Power 19

    Common Titles of Address that indicate Power . 20

    Common Titles of Address that indicate a lack of Power 20

    Examples of Power related Dirty Talk 21

In Relation To Female Genitals 22

    Euphemistic terms that mean Vagina 22

    Dysphemistic terms that mean Vagina 23

    Examples of Female Genitalia Based Dirty Talk .. 24

In Relation To Male Genitals 25

    Euphemistic terms that mean Penis 25

    Dysphemistic terms that mean Penis 26

    Euphemistic terms that mean Testicles 27

    Dysphemistic terms that mean Testicles 27

    Examples of Male Genitalia Based Dirty Talk 28

In Relation To Other Body Parts 29

    Examples of Dirty Talk based on other Body Parts 29

In Relation To Size 30

    Common big adjectives 30

    Common small adjectives 31

    Examples of how Size is implemented into Dirty Talk 31

In Relation to Commands 32

    Examples of Commanding Dirty Talk 33

In Relation To Requests 34

    Examples of Requesting Dirty Talk 34

In Relation To Teasing 35

    Examples of Teasing Dirty Talk 35

In Relation To Compliments 36

    Example of Complimentary Dirty Talk 37

In Relation To Insults 38

Easy Responses 39

    Examples of generic Dirty responses 40

ABOUT THE AUTHOR 41

INTRODUCTION

Are you looking to spice up your love life with some Dirty Talk? Do you want to master the ability to verbally arouse your partner? You've come to the right place.

BDSM is a common occurrence that is practiced by millions of people under different parameters. Many people are first introduced to the concept of BDSM, kinks and fetishes through films, television or social media. This often leads people to having a skewed understanding of the lifestyle, BDSM community and BDSM practices.

Many people believe that BDSM is in someway perverted or outside the realms of 'normal' adult sexual activity. This is not the case however as BDSM can take many different forms. The media often portrays BDSM practitioners as untrustworthy and abusive – this could not be further from the truth. The media portrayal of BDSM often leads people to feel ashamed which leads them to not pursue their BDSM desires. It is perfectly normal and healthy to want to be a Dominant or a Submissive within a BDSM relationship.

It is commonly believed that the relationship between a Submissive and their Dominant has elements of nonconsensual action and that the Submissive will be, constantly or occasionally, forced to act out sexual scenarios and sexually behave in ways they do not desire. It is commonly believed that the Submissive has no power in the relationship and no say on how they are treated. This false idea will be challenged, explained and explored within this book.

Within this book you will find a brief overview of what BDSM actually is and how you can apply it into your relationships. This book also aims to shine a light on many of the common misconceptions held about BDSM, Submissives and Dominants.

So what is BDSM?

BDSM is an initialism for the following: Bondage, Domination (or Discipline), Sadism and Masochism. BDSM is a type of sexual practice that normally involves a couple – but it can be practiced alone or in groups. BDSM will normally include kinks and/or fetishes. BDSM is a mentality that focuses on sensationalizing aspects of sex and will normally include the fusion of pain and pleasure. BDSM normally includes a power relationship – such as that between a Dominant and a Submissive.

What is the difference between a Kink and a Fetish?

It is important to first clarify that the definition of both terms are highly subjective. However within the BDSM community there is a clear difference between a kink and a fetish. A kink is considered to be something that arouses an individual while being outside the sexual norm. This suggests that kinks are subjective and have changed over time. For example holding hands, meeting unchaperoned or kissing with tongues have all been considered kinky in the past but are considered to be utterly normal in modern Western Society. Kinks tend to be more focused on people and actions, such as asphyxiation or domination, whereas fetishes are more focused on specific objects, rituals or specific aspects of an individual's sexuality. A kink is something that an individual highly enjoys but it is not necessary, or even wanted, for every single sex session. A fetish on the other hand is almost always necessary for the person to become sexually aroused. For example someone with a foot fetish will struggle to become aroused unless feet, or shoes, are involved in the sex they are having.

Paraphilias

'Paraphilias' is the term used to describe any sexual

interest that is considered to be atypical. Kinks and fetishes are both considered to be paraphilias. As what is considered to be a paraphilias is based upon what is typical and what is atypical, it suggests that a list of paraphilias will change from culture to culture and will have shifted, changed and evolved throughout history.

Consent, Safety and Safe Words

I'm sure you have all heard the phrase: 'It is better to ask for forgiveness than permission.' This phrase could not be further from truth when it comes to BDSM. The core principles of BDSM is consent, communication and permission. Before engaging into a BDSM relationship, with a Dominant or a Submissive, there should first be a clear conversation about what you are both willing and unwilling to do. What are the limits you both want to impose? What are your turn-ons and turn-offs? What are the safe words? What are your kinks and fetishes? What would you like to explore? What would you like to avoid? It is much safer, healthier and sexually productive to have a conversation outlining what all parties want to gain from the BDSM relationship before actually engaging in the sexual activities. Once boundaries have been discussed, do not cross them. I cannot express enough how important consent, permission and trust are to a happy healthy relationship.

A list of Safe Words

Many aspects of BDSM include restraining, disciplining and punishing. This makes normal safe words (such as 'No,' 'Stop,' and 'Ow') ineffective as they are commonly used during play. It is important to discuss safe words with your partners before engaging in sexual activities to make sure everyone is on the same page. The best Safe Words are short, phonetically identifiable, concise and memorable. Here is a list of example safe words:

- 'Safe word' – There are few instances that someone would utter 'Safe word' during sex which makes it a clear and concise safe word.
- 'Banana' – Words like 'Banana' have a clear phonetic pattern which makes them easily identifiable.
- 'Orange' – Nothing rhymes with orange which makes it a perfect safe word.
- 'Hadron Collider' – Choosing words that are niche, phonetically recognizable and unrelated to sex are a great choice. Other examples of this could be pop culture references, celebrity names, names of children's cartoon characters, names of

subjects you can major in at college and the list goes on.

Non Verbal Safe Words

Being gagged, or restrained, is not an uncommon practice which makes it important to also discuss non-verbal 'Safe words' with your partners. Maybe a specific head movement, hand signal or blinking/tapping pattern could be use.

Traffic Light System

Within the BDSM community, especially during BDSM events, a traffic light system is used to quickly and efficiently gauge people's enjoyment, mentality and consent.

- Green – Green suggests that the person is happy to continue in the play under its current parameters.
- Yellow – Yellow suggests that the person wants to momentarily stop the play to engage in a discussion about the parameters of the paly.
- Red – Red suggests that a predetermined boundary has been crossed and that the person wants to play to stop immediately.

While the traffic light system is simple to use and understand it does have some potential limitations. During some BDSM events the use of the 'Red' safe word is taken very seriously – it will normally lead to all play being halted until the issue is resolved. It suggests that someone has crossed a predetermined boundary. People, usually Doms, who have 'Red' called upon them are normally expelled from and barred from BDSM events. While this hard line stance seems beneficial – it can actually cause a lot of problems. If someone is new to the BDSM scene they may feel uncomfortable using the 'Red' safe word as they do not wish to ruin other people's play or cause their Dom to suffer a social backlash. My perspective on the matter is as follows: if you feel uncomfortable about what is happening to you, it is **imperative** to let your Dom, and the people around you, know. Nothing trumps your own physical and mental wellbeing.

Pain vs. Pleasure

When people imagine the idea of pain and pleasure – they view it in a reductionist form of mere juxtaposition. Everyone has experienced pain and pleasure simultaneously within their life: your mouth burns while eating tasty spicy food, your muscles ache in an accomplished agony after an intense work out. Cognitive neuroscience classifies both pain and pleasure as something known as 'salience'. A salience is an experienced that is important and thereby deserves attention. Salience is fueled by emotion, both positive and negative. When are vices are fulfilled (for example: eating food when hungry, drinking alcohol, having orgasms, intensely working out) our brains release dopamine. When studies are done on pain and pleasure, participants who record the experience as 'most unpleasant' and painful often are noted to release the most amount of dopamine. This suggests that our brains are somewhat hardwired to release dopamine during painful experiences, most likely as a form of coping mechanism. Some people are therefore more likely to derive pleasure from 'painful' experiences.

Common misconceptions about BDSM

A few of the most common misconceptions about BDSM are: that it is unsafe, that is it abusive, that it is immoral and that there is a lot of drug use connected to it. I will know dismantle all of the most common misconceptions. BDSM is asked for, BDSM is not abuse. If two consenting adults wish to 'hurt' each other within the realms of the law – it is not abuse. BDSM is safe, sober and sane. The main mantra of the BDSM community is 'Safe, Sane and Consensual'. When it comes to the idea that BDSM is immoral – I cannot really dispute this idea as what an individual deems to be immoral is based upon their background, upbringing, political views and life experiences. Morality is a complex issue that has been debated since the dawn of humanity – there has yet been a convincing and conclusive answer to the debate. Therefore I argue that BDSM is intrinsically no more, or less, immoral than virtually anything else.

TYPES OF DIRTY TALK

Before we get into the tips and techniques of Dirty Talk, it is first important to note that there are different types of Dirty Talk. The different types of dirty talk include: Playful, Complementary, Degrading and Personal. Each different type of Dirty Talk has different times in which it is most applicable. You might not want to use Degrading Dirty Talk with a partner who is self-conscious. On the other hand, Complementary Dirty Talk should probably be avoided if your partner has a kink for receiving comments of personal degradation.

Playful

Playful Dirty Talk will employ a lot of euphemistic terms and soft phrasing. Playful Dirty Talk will often employ innuendo, inside jokes and playful paralinguistic. Playful Dirty Talk should normally be accompanied with a smile and playful paralinguistic.

Complementary

Complementary Dirty Talk will often involve exaggeration. For example things are: harder, bigger, softer, sweeter, more pleasurable, the best, etc. Complementary Dirty Talk will also exaggerate your emotional response to stimulus. For example: "I love it," rather than "I like it," and "This is the best," rather than "This is good."

Degrading

Degrading Dirty Talk will often involve insults, degrading terms and exaggerating things in a negative manner. For example things are: gross, tiny, disgusting, laughable, a joke, unpleasurable, the worst, etc. Degrading Dirty Talk is normally only used by Dominants towards a Submissive who enjoys personal degradation, humiliation and feeling sexually undesirable.

Personal

Personal Dirty Talk is probably the most effective and arousing type of Dirty Talk. Personal Dirty Talk involves using inside jokes, pet names and other personal names of endearment. Most people find this type of Dirty Talk sexiest because it is based upon the personal relationship and experiences they have shared with their partner.

IN RELATION TO POWER

Power dynamics play an important role in BDSM relationships and sexual relationships as a whole. Power, within the constructs of Dirty Talk, is normally expressed through titles of address. These titles of address can either frame someone as holding power or lacking power. It is important to note that not all powerful terms of address are complimentary, likewise not all powerless terms of address are degrading. Common adjectives that also indicate power are: anything that suggests grandeur, anything that suggests superior size, anything that suggests superior strength and anything that suggests dominance. Common adjectives that also indicate a lack of power are: anything that suggests cheapness or unworthiness, anything that suggests submission, anything that suggests weakness and anything that suggest diminutive sizing.

Common Titles of Address that indicate Power

Below is a list of common terms of address that frame someone as powerful:

- Big One
- Boss
- Captain
- Commander
- Daddy
- Madam
- Master
- Mistress
- Mummy
- Owner
- Sir
- Tyrant
- Your Grace
- Your Highness

Common Titles of Address that indicate a lack of Power

Below is a list of common terms of address that frame someone as powerless:

- Baby
- Boy
- Creature
- Cretin
- Girl
- Little One
- Peasant
- Pet
- Scum
- Servant
- Slave
- Whore
- Worm

Examples of Power related Dirty Talk

"Lick my shoe Slave."

"I'll do whatever you say Mummy."

"I'm Daddy's little whore."

"You're going to be a good Boy now, aren't you?"

"Come give me a backrub, Servant."

"Yes your Highness."

"Anything for you Mistress."

"Yes Sir, I am your little Pet."

"I love feeling owned by you, Your Grace."

"Do you like your little holes being filled by Master?"

"Please fill my unworthy holes Madam."

"Use me like the Scum I am."

"You're going to do exactly what Mummy tells you, or I will have to punish you Little One."

"Get on your knees and be a good little Slave."

IN RELATION TO FEMALE GENITALS

During sex, poetry and loving speech the female genitalia has traditionally been described as delicate, oyster like, flower like and sweet in taste and smell. Qualities that are normally desirable when describing a vagina are: tightness, wetness and warmness.

Euphemistic terms that mean Vagina

Below is a list of common slang terms that are widely accepted and understood to represent the female genitalia in a Euphemistic manner:

- Bearded Clam
- Doodle Sack
- Fancy Bit
- Flower
- Front Bottom
- Fun Tunnel
- Happy Valley
- Hidey Hole
- Hoo-Ha
- Kitty
- Lady Garden
- Lady Parts
- Muffin
- Periwinkle
- Pink Canoe
- Pussy
- Silk Igloo
- South Pole
- Sticky Bun
- Sugar Basin
- Tinkleflower
- Velvet Glove
- Ya-Ya
- Yum-Yum

Dysphemistic terms that mean Vagina

Below is a list of common slang terms that are widely accepted and understood to represent the female genitalia in a Dysphemistic manner:

- Beef Curtains
- Bone Yard
- Cooter
- Cum Dumpster
- Dick Sharpener
- Fish Factory
- Gash
- Knob Gobbler
- Manhole
- Meat Muffin
- Organ Grinder
- Penis Penitentiary
- Pipe Cleaner
- Rocket Pocket
- Sausage Wallet
- Slash
- Slut Muffin
- Snake Charmer
- Tuna Taco
- Vadge

Examples of Female Genitalia Based Dirty Talk

"You have such a tight little pussy."

"Your Kitty always feels so good!"

"Your flower is so sweet and delicate."

"Let me defile your delicate flower."

"I want to lick the pearls from your Oyster."

"I love the taste of your Tuna Taco."

"I want to wear your tight velvet glove."

"I love how warm your Silk Igloo feels on my {fill in the blank}!"

"I can't wait to peel back the petals of your Flower and lick your sweet Rosebud."

"I want to plant my seed inside your Lady Garden."

"Do you want me to butter your Muffin?"

"I love being so deep inside your Sugar Basin."

"Let me ride in your Pink Canoe through your wet rapids."

IN RELATION TO MALE GENITALS

During sex, poetry and loving speech the male genitalia has traditionally been described as strong, snake like, weapon like and musky in taste and smell. Qualities that are normally exaggerated when describing a penis are: size (large is generally preferred), hardness and shape.

Euphemistic terms that mean Penis

Below is a list of common slang terms that are widely accepted and understood to represent the male genitalia in a Euphemistic manner:

- Banana
- Big Boy
- Boner
- Chopper
- Cock
- Dick
- Dong
- Elephant's Trunk
- Hot Dog
- Knob
- Lollipop
- Pecker
- Python
- Rooster
- Sausage
- Snake
- Shaft
- Staff
- Sword
- Trouser Snake

Dysphemistic terms that mean Penis

Below is a list of common slang terms that are widely accepted and understood to represent the male genitalia in a Dysphemistic manner:

- Basilisk
- Boomerang
- Carrot
- Cyclops
- Fuck Stick
- Fuck Truck
- Junk
- Lil' Billy
- Little Boy
- Little Friend
- Little Guy
- Mushroom Tip
- One Eyed Monster
- Prick
- Stick
- Stick Insect
- Turtle Head
- Ugly Thing
- Wang
- Weenie
- Weiner
- Willy
- Worm

Euphemistic terms that mean Testicles

Below is a list of common slang terms that are widely accepted and understood to represent a man's testicles in a Euphemistic manner:

- Balls
- Berries
- Chestnuts
- Coconuts
- Easter Eggs
- Family Jewels
- Golden Globes
- Jellybeans
- Stones
- Walnuts

Dysphemistic terms that mean Testicles

Below is a list of common slang terms that are widely accepted and understood to represent a man's testicles in a Dysphemistic manner:

- Beevis & Butthead
- Coals
- Grenades
- Hairy Hangers
- Itchy & Scratchy
- Meatballs
- Nuts
- Sack
- The Sperm Factory
- The Two Amigos
- Water Balloons
- Weights

Examples of Male Genitalia Based Dirty Talk

"I love your rock hard Cock!"

"You have the biggest dick I've ever seen."

"I love the way your balls taste."

"Put that strong sword inside me."

"I love sucking your lollipop Daddy."

"What a disgusting little worm! Do you really think I would let you put that inside me?"

"I can't wait to drain your water balloons."

"Let me wrap my hands around your huge python."

"I love how hard your Shaft gets for me."

"You're such a dirty boy with a little Fuck Stick."

"Let me wake that Little Guy up for you."

"Let me wake that Big Boy up for you."

"Your Hot Dog stretches my mouth so nicely."

"I want your big, hard, throbbing Trouser Snake inside me more than anything."

IN RELATION TO OTHER BODY PARTS

There are multiple other body parts that could be the subject of Dirty Talking. There are a lot of common fetishes that revolve around different body parts such as: hair fetishes, breast fetishes, foot fetishes, tongue fetishes and hand fetishes. When including a body part within your Dirty Talk it is important to use adjectives and lexical devices that are appropriate to the body part. For example it is perfectly normal to describe a tongue as 'wet' but describing a foot as 'wet' is less appropriate.

Examples of Dirty Talk based on other Body Parts

"Your tongue is so long and wet."

"You have such delicate feet."

"I love your strong hands"

"I love your soft silken breasts."

"Rub your dirty tongue here."

"I love worshiping your unclean feet."

"Let me suck on your pretty fingers."

"Do you like how I pull your hair?"

IN RELATION TO SIZE

Size is an important aspect of most couple's Dirty Talk. As previously mentioned men are generally referred to as big, wide and strong and women are referred to as small, tight and delicate. However these normalities do not apply to **ALL** relationships. For example if someone is into Big Beautiful Women, the use of adjectives like 'big' and 'giant' are highly applicable and the general adjectives of 'small' and 'tiny' are not appropriate. You should try to filter your use of size based Dirty Talk on who your partner is, what your partner wants and what the parameters of your BDSM relationship are.

Common big adjectives

Below is a list of common adjectives used to describe the largeness of a partner, or parts of a partner, during sex:

- Big
- Epic
- Giant
- Girthy
- Great
- Huge
- Immense
- Large
- Massive
- Monstrous
- Voluptuous
- Wide

Common small adjectives

Below is a list of common adjectives used to describe the smallness of a partner, or parts of a partner, during sex:

- Baby
- Dinky
- Little
- Mini
- Petite
- Pocket Sized
- Small
- Tight
- Tiny
- Wee

Examples of how Size is implemented into Dirty Talk

"I love your big cock."

"You have such a pretty little pussy."

"Your curves are so voluptuous."

"I cant get enough of your tight mouth."

"You have such a long tongue."

"I love your petite boobs."

"I love your mini dick."

IN RELATION TO COMMANDS

Commands are an important aspect of BDSM as they are a clear indication of one party's power over the other. Commands also allow a Submissive to disobey, which generally leads to punishment. Commands allow a Submissive to feel out of control while also allowing a Dominant to feel in control. It is important to discuss which activities should be commanded and which activities should be requested within the parameters of your BDSM relationship. It is important to note that Submissive's can also command their Dominants – but commands are generally made by Dominants.

When using commands it is important to try and include imperatives. An imperative command is defined by its importance and the authority behind it. The main difference between a command and a request is the phrasing. A request will nearly always be constructed as a question. For example: "Can you get on your knees?" Commands will never be phrased as questions. For example: "Get on your knees."

Examples of Commanding Dirty Talk

"Get on your Knees."

"Cum for me."

"Eat my pussy."

"Suck my dick."

"Fuck me harder. Fuck me faster."

"Choke me."

"Undress for me."

"Tell me how good that feels."

"Tell me how much you like that!"

"Don't cum yet – I'm not finished with you."

"Look at me while I fuck you."

"Spread that ass for me."

"Get into {insert desired sexual position}."

"Keep going! That feels amazing."

"Open your mouth and suck on my fingers."

"Lick my Clit more gently."

IN RELATION TO REQUESTS

Requests are the Submissive's version of a command. Requests allow a Submissive to still feel out of control. As previously mentioned, the main difference between a request and a command is the phrasing. Commands will always state "Do this." Requests can be questions or suggest that you want someone to do something – for example "Please do this," or "Could you do this."

Examples of Requesting Dirty Talk

"I need you inside me now, please Sir."

"Let me take control tonight?"

"Could you suck my dick a little longer?"

"Do you want me to make you come?"

"Please can you fuck me harder?"

"I want you to dominant me Daddy."

"Have I been a good little {insert preferred term of sexual address}."

"Please don't stop."

IN RELATION TO TEASING

Teasing is an important aspect of BDSM relationships. The anticipation of sexual gratification generally leads to more intense orgasms and more intense sex. Teasing Dirty Talk can be used during foreplay or well in advance of sex. Teasing can also be used in orgasm-denial as a further way to increase the intensity of your partner's orgasm.

Examples of Teasing Dirty Talk

"I am not going to let you Cum until you beg me."

"I won't stop {insert sexual activity} until you are about to burst."

"I'm too busy tonight, so you will have to wait until tomorrow."

"You're going to have to show me how much you want it."

"I thought of new something that I want to try with you tonight."

"I'm going to tease you all night until you're nice and wet/hard for me."

"I'm going to tease you till you can't stand it!"

IN RELATION TO COMPLIMENTS

Compliments are an important part of Dirty Talk, BDSM relationships and most other relationships a person will experience throughout their life. Compliments indicate your interest in your partner. Compliments can also be used as a great way to subtly command your partner to continue what they are doing. Compliments can also be a great way of encouraging your partner if they are nervous, are new to the type of play you are initiating or are sexually inexperienced. Compliments are also a fantastic way of stroking your partner's ego and making them more aroused, committed to proving your compliment to be correct and making them more confident in themselves and their sexual prowess.

When giving compliments during sex it is useful to sometimes try to exaggerate what you are feeling and how well your partner is performing. I suggest using superlatives during complementary Dirty Talk to achieve this. No matter what the adjective is, or the context in which it is being used, a superlative will always leave your partner feeling like they are the best.

Example of Complimentary Dirty Talk

"You make me the wettest I've ever been."

"You make my dick harder than I thought possible."

"Your body makes me so horny."

"You have the prettiest {fill in the blank}."

"I love the way your {fill in the blank} makes me feel."

"I can't control myself when I'm around you."

"I can't get over how amazingly {insert adjective} your {insert body part} is."

"I can't get enough of you!"

"No one is as good as you at that."

"I've never cum like this before! You're a sex god/goddess."

"You've made me cum more than I thought was possible."

"I've never felt anything this good in my whole life."

IN RELATION TO INSULTS

While compliments are an everyday occurrence within most relationships – insults are definitely a rarer occurrence. Insults used during sex are even more niche. Insulting Dirty Talk should only be used when your partner has a kink for personal degradation or when you are trying to misbehave to receive punishment. One of the most effective ways to insult your partner is through degrading adjectives and degrading terms of address.

Before using insulting Dirty Talk it is important to understand how your partner will respond. You do not want to ruin your sexual moment by upsetting your partner.

Examples of Degrading Terms of Address

Below is a list of Degrading Terms of Address:

- Bitch
- Cow
- Cretin
- Cunt
- Dick
- Maggot
- Mistake
- Monster
- Peasant
- Pig
- Prick
- Slag
- Slut
- Wanker
- Whore
- Worm

Examples of Insulting Dirty Talk

"You're such a disgusting Mistake."

"Who would ever want to touch you? You're the dirtiest little piggy with the smallest dick in town."

"You're such an ugly slut."

"It's a shame such a big Dick, like yourself, has such a tiny dick."

"You aren't even worthy of licking my shoes, you filthy unwanted Cretin."

"I've never seen such a gross Slag in my life."

"You're such a pathetic little Worm."

"You're nothing but a brain dead Cow."

"You make my physically sick Maggot."

"Why am I wasting my time with a Prick like you?"

"You're lucky I'm kind enough to even touch you, you dirty little Wanker."

"Your Peasant hands are not worthy of touching my majesty."

"Do you like being my Whore?"

EASY RESPONSES

Some times your partner will prompt you to talk Dirty and you won't be able to think of a sexy response. Sometimes you will be too focused on sex, punishment or another aspect of BDSM to be able to quickly think of a contextual response. Sometimes you won't feel especially dirty but don't want to disappoint your partner. If you've ever experienced any of the above scenarios – don't worry, it is perfectly normal.

Dirty Talk should always be a fun activity for you and your partner to enjoy. It allows you to express your desires, emotions and what you are feeling in a creative and sexy way. Dirty Talk generally has no parameters – and if parameters are needed, they should be discussed well in advance of you engaging in any sexual activity.

If you are having trouble with Dirty Talking this section is definitely for you! Below is a list of responses that will keep the passion in your play. This list should serve you well in, almost, any sexual context.

Examples of generic Dirty responses

"I love how you feel."

"I love how you fuck me."

"You fuck me so good."

"Yes! Give me more of that {insert appropriate genitals]."

"That turns me on so much!"

"What else do you want to do to me?"

"I'm all yours."

"I love it when you talk Dirty to me."

"It feels so good – I can barely think of what to say."

"You're blowing my mind."

"Don't stop."

"Yes {inset whatever name you generally call your partner during sex]."

"You're the best at this."

"No one makes me cum as hard as you."

Maxwell Diamond

ABOUT THE AUTHOR

My name is Maxwell. I have been a member of the BDSM community on and off for the last 12 years and have been a committed member of the scene for the last 6 years. During my sexual history I have been a Dominant, a Submissive and a Switch. I have witnessed and taken part in a wide variety of play – from spanking to shibari. While I am passionate about the BDSM community, I am more so passionate about spreading awareness about consent and the importance of physical wellbeing and mental wellbeing in the sexual realm. BDSM has changed my life. It has given me confidence, it has lead to some of the most valuable friendships in my life and through BDSM I have found my long term partner.

Life is short. Lead the sexual life you desire and deserve.

Maxwell Diamond

BDSM: Dirty Talk 101

Made in United States
North Haven, CT
21 January 2022